HOW TO RELIEVE PAIN, ANXIETY AND STRESS WITH CBD OIL WITHOUT SIDE EFFECTS IN 1 DAY

TABLE OF CONTENTS

INTRODUCTION

Stress, anxiety and chronic pain are symptoms that more and more people are suffering from in these modern times. Work conditions are often responsible for many of these symptoms. However, other things such as medical conditions, prescrip tion drugs and day-to-day struggles can also cause an otherwise healthy person to suffer from these issues. What many people are looking for is relief in the form of something that is safe, easy to use and inexpensive. Recent medical and scientific studies suggest that Cannabidiol, otherwise known as CBD oil, might just be the answer. Not only is it cheap and easy to use, CBD oil also has few side-effects, all of which are mild to moderate in nature. Furthermore, CBD lacks the mind-altering effects of THC, making it a more socially acceptable compound found in the cannabis plant.

All in all, CBD has been found to be a non-addictive, harmless and effective treatment for things such as chronic pain, headaches, high blood pressure, stress and anxiety symptoms and a whole range of other conditions that affect millions of people around the world. This book will discuss the healing properties of CBD oil, along with how it works and in what forms it is available. Additionally, the few side-effects associated with CBD will be discussed, along with ways to effectively counter them. By the time you finish reading this book you will know whether or not CBD oil has the potential of helping you to eliminate the symptoms you suffer from, thereby restoring you to the happy and stress-free life you so richly deserve!

CHAPTER 1: WHAT IS CBD OIL?

CBD oil is something that has gained both popularity and notoriety within the medical community in recent years. Many research studies have shown promising results regarding the healing properties of CBD oil. However, some scientists remain skeptical, largely due to the legal complications of the product. Nevertheless, enough evidence has surfaced to suggest that CBD oil, when used properly, can help a person to manage pain, stress, and a whole host of other conditions and symptoms that would otherwise require stronger medications that are potentially dangerous and even addictive. Before exploring the healing properties of CBD oil, it is important to discuss what it actually is. This chapter will present the basic information of CBD oil without getting too heavily involved in the science, thus making it easier for the average person to fully understand.

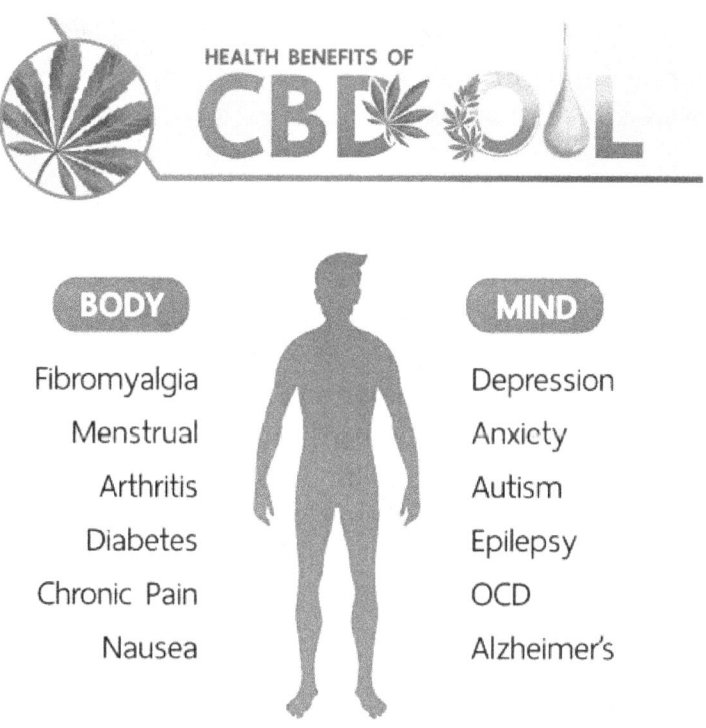

Where CBD oil comes from

The first step to understanding CBD oil is to know its origin. CBD oil, otherwise known as Cannabidiol, is a substance found in the cannabis plant. Unfortunately, this has caused numerous problems, both in terms of legal issues as well as moral and ethical issues. This is because cannabis is one of the most controversial plants on the planet, most commonly associated with marijuana and the stigma attached to its use. However, CBD oil is not and should not be associated with smoking a joint as it is not a part of the process of "getting high." Instead, it is a perfectly harmless chemical compound that has numerous health benefits, both in terms of physical health as well as mental health. Only when this separation is fully understood can CBD oil be addressed in a fair and impartial manner, allowing it the attention it truly deserves.

While CBD oil can be found in cannabis plants cultivated for marijuana production, most of it actually comes from the more innocuous cannabis plants used for hemp production. The truth of the matter is that most marijuana specific plants have been genetically manipulated in order to increase THC content. As a result, CBD levels are usually lower in these plants, making them less capable of producing any significant quantities of CBD oil. In contrast, hemp producing plants maintain the higher levels of CBD that are naturally occurring in cannabis plants. Therefore, most of the CBD oil found on the market today can be traced to hemp plants, not the socially shunned marijuana plants. This affects both the moral and legal aspects of CBD, as it is produced from legal plants in professional environments. Unfortunately, there are still many people who fail to separate the different types of cannabis plant, let alone the different compounds found within. Subsequently, CBD oil is still highly restricted in certain states as well as certain countries around the world.

CBD vs. THC

When anyone hears the term "cannabis" they doubtlessly envision such things as marijuana smoking hippies or college students passing around a joint while listening to the Grateful Dead. While these images do have some merit they hardly present the full picture of cannabis. In fact, they don't even present the full picture of marijuana and its use. In order to get a proper perspective on this it is necessary to understand what makes marijuana impact users the way it does.

The feeling of "getting high" that comes from smoking or ingesting marijuana is a result of the THC levels. THC, otherwise known as Tetrahydrocannabinol, is a chemical compound found within the cannabis plant. It is the element that makes a person feel super relaxed and sleepy when smoking marijuana. This feeling is what is known as a psychoactive effect, something that directly affects how a person's mind functions. Cannabis plants bred for marijuana production have been genetically altered to increase THC levels, usually resulting in lower CBD levels as a result. This creates a product that provides the mental experience without the actual benefits that CBD oil offers.

In contrast, CBD oil provides a whole range of physical and mental benefits, all without the psychoactive properties of THC. This difference is what underlies the two variations of marijuana — medical and recreational. Recreational marijuana is the strain that contains high levels of THC and low levels of CBD. Alternatively, medical marijuana has higher levels of CBD and lower levels of THC. While it might seem reasonable to try to eliminate the THC altogether the simple fact is that CBD is more effective when used in balance with THC. Therefore, medical marijuana still contains levels of THC, just not the same levels that are found in the marijuana being passed around in the college dorm. Unfortunately, it is because of this that the issue of legalizing medical marijuana is still such a contentious one, preventing people from enjoying the medical benefits that CBD oil can provide when used in its most natural form. Fortunately, CBD oil can be used on its own to a significant effect, and that is what this book is going to reveal.

CHAPTER 2: HOW CBD OIL WORKS

Knowing where CBD oil comes from and the difference between it and THC is only half of the bigger picture. The other half is in knowing how CBD actually works. It isn't enough to simply say "take two of these and you'll feel better." Instead, you need to know exactly how and why CBD oil can treat and cure the conditions it has been proven to be effective against. This chapter will address the scientific reasons behind the effectiveness of CBD oil, albeit in a way that allows a person without a Ph.D. to understand the information provided. Additionally, this chapter will discuss how the body works when it comes to such things as stress, pain and other negative conditions. By understanding both of these aspects you will be able to make a far more educated decision when it comes to deciding whether or not CBD oil is right for you.

The Endocannabinoid System (ECS)

In order to understand just how CBD oil has the effects that it does it is necessary to understand how the body functions. Any time a person experiences pain it is considered a purely physical phenomenon, usually attributed to an external stimulus. In other words, if you hit your finger with a hammer you blame the hammer for the pain you feel. While this is true to a degree there is, in fact, a whole other dimension as to why you actually feel pain when you experience a trauma. This dimension is the chemical interaction within the body. Any time your body experiences trauma it sends signals to the brain, which in turn releases the chemical histamine. In superficial traumas, such as a bug bite or skin abrasion histamine will cause an itching sensation. However, in deeper traumas histamine will actually cause the sensation of pain. This is the body's way of alerting you to the trauma, just in case you didn't realize you hit your finger with the hammer!

Such chemical reactions aren't limited to pain and itchiness. Instead, they underlie every physical and mental sensation a person experience. These include such things as hunger, fear, anger and even love. The bottom line is that emotions, feelings and the like are all chemically induced experiences, created by the brain and other chemical producing organs within the body. Most of the time these chemicals are produced in carefully calculated levels, providing just enough of a response to get the point across. This balance is what is referred to as homeostasis, the state of all physical and mental processes being in perfect equilibrium. Unfortunately, sometimes this balance is interrupted, creating unhealthy levels of fear, pain or even pleasure depending on the specific chemical being over or under produced. This is where the Endocannabinoid System (ECS) comes into play.

The ECS is a system that was discovered relatively recently, beginning in 1988. Studies on animals determined the existence of cannabinoid receptors, which were responsible for maintaining the proper levels of chemical production within the body. Later studies revealed that these receptors were also present within humans. Two main receptors were determined to be responsible for chemicals that affected the body and the brain respectively. As the name might suggest, these receptors were activated by ingestion of the cannabis plant. This is where CBD and THC come into play. While THC largely affects the mind, CBD influences chemicals that affect both physical and mental health. When CBD is administered to a subject experiencing pain the result is that the production of histamines responsible for the pain is reduced.

Furthermore, natural chemicals that fight pain, such as serotonin or norepinephrine, are increased, thus providing pain relief to the individual.

Rather than being seen as a miracle drug, CBD should be understood as having the very same impact than any other drug has. Any time you take an aspirin or an allergy medication you are ingesting compounds that impact the chemical production within your body. Aspirin doesn't actually kill pain, rather it reduces the pain chemicals while helping to release pain killing chemicals. This is the same function that CBD serves. The main difference is that CBD influences a whole system within the human body designed for cannabinoid reception. Therefore, it can be seen as a truly natural and homeopathic way to treat and cure conditions that would otherwise require harmful and potentially addictive medications.

Effects of CBD oil

The impact of CBD oil on the homeostasis of an individual simply cannot be overstated. Not only does this help to reduce and even eliminate pain, it can also impact such things as appetite disorders, stress, anxiety, sleep disorders and even depression. Again, CBD oil isn't some magical potion that contains all sorts of "fix-it" drugs, rather it is a natural compound that helps to regulate chemical production within the human body. Any time a person suffers from insomnia or fatigue it is the result of too little or too much melatonin being produced. CBD simply restores this production to proper levels, thereby allowing a person to get the right amount of sleep and live a productive and healthy life. The same thing applies to appetite disorders. Being too hungry or not hungry enough is the result of a chemical imbalance. Once the imbalance is corrected the individual will experience a proper appetite cycle once again. The Endocannabinoid System is designed to perform this very function. Therefore, taking CBD oil is a sure way to correct a symptom or condition that is the direct consequence of a chemical imbalance.

Restoring healthy chemical production levels can provide even greater benefits than you might imagine. This is particularly true in the case of anxiety. When the body becomes stressed it produces cortisol, which influences the body and mind in times of perceived threat. An increase in blood pressure, mental awareness and other important physiological and psychological functions help a person to find the energy and stamina to face an immediate challenge. While this is good in proper amounts, too much cortisol can cause such things as stress, high blood pressure, and even mental instability. Rage and phobia related emotions can also be a result of unregulated cortisol production. By restoring balance to cortisol production, CBD will not only lower blood pressure and reduce the emotional symptoms of anxiety, it will also restore the mind to a proper level of calm, taking it off of the "high alert" condition that cortisol puts it on. This allows a person to actually perceive events in a different way, seeing things as less threatening than a mind influenced by high levels of cortisol. Thus, not only can CBD reduce the effects of stress, it can help a person to see life in a more normal way as well, virtually preventing stress as a result.

Finally, the actual chemical properties of CBD oil need to be considered in order to fully appreciate the benefits it can have for a person suffering from pain or stress related symptoms. CBD possesses anti-inflammatory properties, making it a natural pain reliever. Since inflammation is often associated with pain, anything that reduces swelling will also go a long way to reducing the pain as well. Therefore, in addition to regulating chemical production within the body, CBD can have a direct influence on pain as well. The same can be said for stress. CBD has been classified as an anti-anxiolytic, meaning that it provides stress relief when taken. Thus, as well as regulating the production of stress-causing chemicals CBD can also directly reduce stress, thereby providing relief from multiple directions.

CHAPTER 3: CBD OIL AND PAIN

Of all the benefits associated with CBD oil, perhaps the most significant is that of pain management. This is true both in terms of medical research and personal accounts. Numerous studies have shown CBD oil to be highly effective when it comes to reducing and even eliminating pain. Part of this is due to the effect that CBD has on the production of chemicals as already stated in this book. The other end of this has to do with the anti-inflammatory properties of CBD. However, if you want proof that CBD oil has the ability to beat even the most chronic and stubborn of pains you don't have to rely on scientific research, instead you can simply examine the countless cases where people who couldn't find relief with traditional medicines were suddenly pain-free once they started using CBD oil on a regular basis. This chapter will examine the different types of pain that CBD reportedly is capable of eliminating, as well as the proper methods for using CBD oil, thereby enabling you to know how to start using CBD oil to treat your symptoms.

Types of pain treatable with CBD oil

One of the most common forms of pain experienced by adults is that of joint pain. The reason for this is that joint pain affects both those who suffer from specific conditions as well as those who are fairly healthy overall. A person only needs to wear the wrong type of shoes or stand on their feet all day in order to suffer pain in their knees. Elbow pain is equally common, especially among those who play sports such as tennis, golf and the like. Subsequently, millions of adults around the world experience joint pain in one form or another on a fairly regular basis.

Fortunately, CBD oil can help to make all the difference, reducing not only the pain symptoms, but also reducing the very cause of the pain itself. This is because it has the ability to reduce the swelling that can be at the heart of joint pain. Needless to say, the anti-inflammatory quality of CBD oil is particularly effective when it comes to arthritis. Since arthritis is the number one cause of joint pain among adults, this makes CBD oil a virtual godsend, seeing as it can reduce the swelling and eliminate the pain without the cost or danger associated with traditional arthritic pain medications.

Another type of pain common in adults around the world is back pain. This usually comes in the form of lower back pain, caused by a wide range of factors. Standing on hard floors for long periods of time, wearing shoes with little arch support, having a bad mattress and heavy manual labor are just a few examples of these factors. Unfortunately, almost every adult comes face to face with one or more of these conditions on an almost daily basis, resulting in chronic back pain. While there are numerous pain relief medications on the market that are designed to reduce back pain most of these have been shown to have harmful side effects, effects that are often as bad as if not worse than the back pain itself. Fortunately, CBD oil can reduce and even eliminate back pain without any of these harmful side effects. Furthermore, the body won't develop a tolerance to CBD oil the way that it will to stronger drugs. This means that the dose you use now is the same dose that you will need to relieve your pain ten years from now.

Muscle pain is the third type of pain commonly treated with CBD oil. Some forms of muscle pain can be attributed to strain or mild trauma which can cause muscle and tissue inflammation. Again, the anti-inflammatory quality of CBD oil makes it highly effective in not only treating this type of pain but also eliminating the very cause altogether. However, muscle pain can also be the result of more serious conditions, including such things as Parkinson's disease, multiple sclerosis and other incurable muscle conditions. The good news is that CBD oil can actually help to significantly reduce pain in these cases, as well as reducing muscle spasms caused by these and other similar conditions.

This is more than merely word of mouth. Numerous studies conducted over the past several years have revealed that CBD oil is highly effective in treating the symptoms of Parkinson's, multiple sclerosis and the like. In some studies pain was reduced by a full third or more, while muscle spasms were reduced by a full fifty percent. Although this is a long way from the cure that CBD oil can provide for less severe conditions it is considered nothing short of a miracle. This is largely due to the fact that no conventional drug can provide such significant relief without causing a whole host of dangerous and devastating side effects. Furthermore, CBD oil is considerably cheaper than these more dangerous drugs, making it a better choice all around.

How, when and how much to take

As with any medication it is vital that you know exactly how, when and how much to take in order to achieve the maximum benefits possible. The first rule of thumb is to always consult a proper medical doctor before taking any type of medication, CBD oil included. This will help to ensure that you won't experience any side effects that can occur if you are taking other medications or supplements. Fortunately, very few side effects have been reported with the use of CBD oil, and those that have been reported are usually fairly minor and safe.

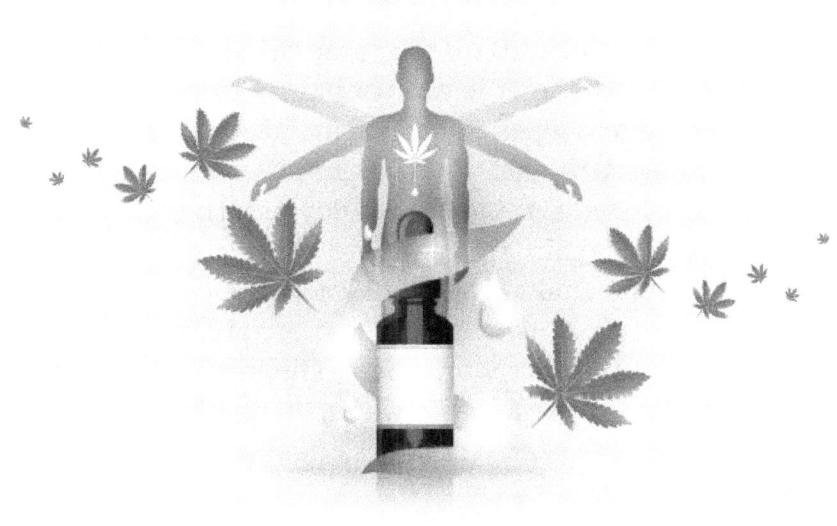

When it comes to the 'how,' CBD oil comes in different forms in order to tackle different pains and ailments. Topical cream, for example, is the number one choice for anyone suffering muscle or lower back pain. This can also be an effective form when it comes to joint pain as you can apply the cream directly to your knee, shoulder or elbow and begin to experience the pain relief right away. Other forms include smokables, edibles, capsules, patches and drops. Some of these forms are designed to deliver CBD oil more effectively to the target area, whereas others are designed for convenience. Smoking, for example, may be an effective way to ingest CBD. However, it is not always permitted and in some cases is even illegal. Drops are more convenient, but it can take longer for them to take effect. A good way to determine what works for you is through trial and error. By trying different forms, you can discover which ones your body responds to best. Additionally, you can choose to use several forms simultaneously. In this case you can use cream or drops during the day, especially if you are at work and are restricted with regards to smoking and the like. At night, however, when such restrictions are no longer relevant, you can use smokables, edibles or any other form that has a more effective impact on your pain or discomfort.

As far as when to take CBD oil the same principles will apply as when taking any other medication or pain regimen. Some people will choose to take it when the pain flairs up, or at more demanding times of day. Alternatively, they might wish to introduce a steady dose of CBD all throughout the day, as is the case with most pain medications. Again, this is where consulting with a doctor can be highly beneficial as they will know the best approach for your specific needs. However, trial and error can also go a long way to determining what works best. The important thing is to recognize that CBD isn't a magic wand, instead it is a pain treatment and should be taken with the same discipline as any other pain medication.

Doses differ depending on the form and strength of the CBD oil. Lower doses will prove effective for minor and temporary pains, while stronger doses will be more beneficial for chronic and severe pain management. The most common dose is 25mg, twice a day. This can be taken in any form. However, capsules and drops are usually the best way to ensure an accurate dose. Taken first thing in the morning and midway through the day will help to provide the strongest pain relief during your most demanding times of day. It is recommended that you follow this dosage for a full three weeks in order to build the levels in your body. If you still struggle with pain or discomfort after three weeks you might choose to increase the dose or the number of times you take CBD during the day. Again, allow a full three weeks after any change to determine the full impact of the change. Fortunately, you don't have to worry about any dangers when it comes to trying to find the right dose for you. CBD is not addictive, and there is no known case of someone overdosing on it. Even so, you should consider getting advice from a medical professional while determining the right CBD regimen for you.

CHAPTER 4: EFFECTS OF CBD OIL ON STRESS AND ANXIETY

Physical pain isn't the only type of pain treated by CBD oil. Numerous studies, as well as countless personal accounts reveal how CBD oil can also help to treat and cure mental and emotional distress. In fact, everything from mood swings to full on post-traumatic stress disorder have been shown to be significantly impacted by regular and responsible use of CBD oil. This is a huge breakthrough, especially for anyone who wants to treat their depression or anxiety symptoms without the highly addictive medications currently prescribed by doctors. While some may remain skeptical of the effectiveness of CBD oil for such things as depression and anxiety it has actually been approved by the Food and Drug Administration for such applications. This means that the government has been convinced by the results of scientific and medical studies, leaving little room for the doubters and naysayers. This chapter will cover some of the more common emotional and mental conditions treatable with CBD oil, thereby helping you to decide whether or not this form of treatment might be right for you.

Types of stress and anxiety treatable with CBD oil

Anyone who has struggled with stress or anxiety will know just how great of an impact they can have on a person's life. Furthermore, they will understand that there are numerous forms of stress and anxiety, some being easy to identify while others can be misidentified and even overlooked entirely. As a result, finding the right medication, let alone the proper dosage, can be a monumental challenge. Fortunately, CBD oil makes this process easier as it addresses the causes of most stress and anxiety conditions in a gentle yet effective way.

One form of anxiety that is virtually cured with CBD oil is that of social anxiety. Most people have social anxiety to one degree or another, but few feel the need to engage in costly and dangerous medications to overcome their symptoms. In some cases, a person will be OK in most social situations, only feeling significant levels of anxiety in the case of public speaking or other such situations, which see them in the proverbial spotlight. Alternatively, others feel anxious simply being in large crowds or having to engage in conversation with perfect strangers, such as at a coffee shop or the checkout line in the grocery store. No matter how serious the symptoms, CBD oil can help to regulate the chemical reaction to social anxiety, thereby restoring peace of mind and a healthy social life.

This same regulation of chemical reactions in the brain is how CBD oil combats the more serious conditions of depression and post-traumatic stress disorder. Needless to say, such conditions, especially in the case of PTSD, should never be dismissed as merely chemical imbalances. However, it is these imbalances that significantly amplify the symptoms suffered by the individual. Therefore, when chemical balances in the brain are restored the symptoms are reduced if not eliminated, thus allowing a person to live a normal life in spite of the traumas that they have had to endure. One of the main chemicals that influence depression and PTSD is serotonin. CBD oil has been scientifically proven to restore serotonin production to healthy levels, thus reducing if not eliminating such things as lethargy, paranoia, fatigue and other symptoms of depression and anxiety. Again, the simple and safe nature of CBD oil makes it a hugely popular alternative over medications that can cause serious, if not deadly side effects.

Another common condition treatable with CBD oil is what is known as Generalized Anxiety Disorder (GAD). This is often mistaken for regular stress though it is, in fact, a more serious condition. Someone suffering from GAD will demonstrate stress and anxiety in every situation in their life. They will often worry excessively about things that aren't really important, or they will create scenarios to worry about, scenarios that are usually fairly unrealistic and thus not reasonable causes for concern. One of the main causes for GAD is a chemical imbalance in the brain, often associated with high levels of salivary cortisol. When CBD oil is administered to a person suffering from GAD the homeostatic nature of it helps bring cortisol production to normal levels, thus eliminating the symptoms of anxiety caused by too much cortisol. Not only does this make the individual feel better, it also enables them to approach their life with a clear mind, thus allowing them to handle any serious issues with greater effect.

Finally, there is the condition of general stress, one that is experienced by virtually everyone at some point in their life if not on a regular basis. This is characterized by feeling anxious about such things as financial security, job security and other day to day events that could prove disastrous if they were to go wrong. Anyone with a stressful job will experience these anxieties on a more regular basis. However, everyone will have some event or situation come along that will cause them to feel anxious as to their overall wellbeing. These symptoms are the perfectly natural side effects of the increased cortisol production that takes place during stressful moments. Ordinarily, such symptoms are relatively mild and go away once circumstances return to normal. However, in the event that stressful conditions are long-lasting some form of relief is often required to keep symptoms from spiraling out of control. CBD oil can provide this relief by keeping chemical production in the brain regulated, thereby helping a person to remain mentally and emotionally strong and healthy during unusually stressful situations.

CHAPTER 5: OTHER BENEFITS OF CBD OIL

In addition to treating a wide range of conditions related to stress and anxiety, CBD oil can help treat numerous other neurological and physiological symptoms. Many of these symptoms are the harmful side-effects of prescription medications used for serious illnesses. The things that make CBD oil so remarkable in this case is that it can be mixed with virtually any other medication without fear of complications, which is something, most prescription drugs cannot claim. Therefore, not only can CBD oil provide relief from mild or severe symptoms, it can do so without causing any further harm to the individual's body and mind, and for a fraction of the cost of the traditional medications that can prove more harmful than the conditions they are treating.

Other physiological conditions treatable with CBD oil

Perhaps the most notable of the conditions treatable with CBD oil are the side effects of cancer treatment. Chemotherapy, although a proven treatment for cancer, is a highly aggressive regimen that wreaks havoc on a person's body. Pain, nausea and insomnia are just a few of the common side-effects of this treatment. While there are numerous drugs available to fight these symptoms, many fails to produce meaningful results for most cancer patients. Furthermore, the addition of strong medications during chemotherapy can create added risks, seeing as the body is in a more vulnerable state due to the chemo drugs. Since CBD oil is a natural chemical, one that the body is designed to process, it makes sense that it should be used in such a delicate situation as chemotherapy. Not only does it help to regulate the natural chemicals in the brain, it also has been shown to significantly reduce such symptoms as nausea, pain and insomnia, thereby bringing welcome relief to cancer patients all over the world. Perhaps the best thing about CBD oil is that it can be used in conjunction with other medications, thus increasing their effectiveness. Therefore, a person can choose to use traditional drugs to fight chemotherapy side-effects and add CBD oil to increase the results.

In addition to reducing the side-effects of cancer treatments, CBD oil has in fact also been demonstrated to fight cancer directly. Studies in Britain showed that CBD helped to prevent cancer from spreading by suppressing the growth of cancer cells. Additionally, some studies showed CBD to actually aid in the destruction of cancer cells, thus helping to eliminate it altogether. One theory behind these results is that CBD is able to combat cancer cell generation by reducing the toxicity levels in a person's body. Cancer is more common in people with higher levels of toxicity, therefore anything that lowers toxic levels can reduce and even prevent cancer in the first place. Further research is being conducted to collect more data regarding the cancer fighting potential of CBD, however, the early results do seem very promising.

One of the words most commonly used when referring to the properties of CBD oil is "regulating." While this word may seem far less impactful than words such as "cure" or "prevention" it should not be underestimated. The simple fact is that most medical conditions are the result of imbalances of one form or another. For example, heart disease is usually the result of high blood pressure. Therefore, anything that can help to "regulate" blood pressure can have a profound impact on heart disease itself. CBD oil has been shown to do just that. By regulating a person's blood pressure, a CBD regimen can virtually eliminate the symptoms of heart disease, thus being the next best thing to an actual cure. Likewise, the same can be said for diabetes. By regulating the sugar levels in a person, CBD oil can eliminate the symptoms of diabetes, thus allowing someone with the disease to live a normal and healthy life. While results can differ from person to person, studies have proven definitively that using CBD oil will improve the health and wellbeing of a person suffering from such things as heart disease or diabetes.

CBD oil isn't just for symptoms attributed to such extreme conditions as Alzheimer's and diabetes. The fact of the matter is that it can reduce or even eliminate a whole host of mild to moderate conditions as well. One such condition that has been impacted in numerous medical studies is that of acne. Since acne has a wide range of causes it isn't guaranteed that CBD oil will eliminate it for everyone. However, it has been shown effective in cases where acne was caused by hormonal imbalances or inflammatory conditions. This stands to reason given the fact that the two main attributes of CBD are its anti-inflammatory and regulatory properties. That CBD oil is both safe and non-addictive means that it can be used by people of all ages, provided that such use is legal and recommended by a medical professional. Furthermore, since acne is a skin condition the CBD oil can be applied as a cream, making it both perfectly safe and easy to use.

Other neurological conditions treatable with CBD oil

The anti-inflammatory properties of CBD oil have been shown to reduce and even prevent neurodegeneration caused by such diseases as Alzheimer's. As a result, the cognitive decline associated with Alzheimer's disease was virtually prevented, enabling a person with the disease to live a more normal life far beyond what is normal in most cases. This doesn't mean that CBD oil cures Alzheimer's, rather it means that it reduces and even prevents the damage that Alzheimer's causes. While studies are still being conducted in this area the early results have been highly positive, suggesting that CBD oil may, in fact, be the next best thing to a cure for anyone suffering such debilitating diseases.

Another effective application for CBD has been found in the area of addiction recovery. Anyone who has tried to break any habit or addiction will know of the untold stress such changes can bring. More often than not this stress will cause a person to return to the habit or addiction, undoing all of the progress they had previously made. Due to its ability to reduce symptoms of stress and anxiety, CBD has been proven to help people overcome all sorts of addictions. The most notable addictions more easily broken with the use of CBD were smoking and opioid use. However, the mood regulating and pain reducing qualities of CBD make it helpful in virtually any addiction recovery, giving a person an invaluable edge in fighting their reliance on substances of any kind.

CHAPTER 6: HOW TO AVOID SIDE EFFECTS OF CBD OIL

Since research on the effects of CBD oil is still in its early stages there is a lack of sufficient data to indicate whether or not there are significant side-effects related to its use. One thing that is clear is that no serious symptoms have ever been experienced, meaning that the use of CBD oil is considered safe within all research studies. There are, however, a few mild to moderate side-effects that have shown up among several users, enough to suggest that CBD oil is not altogether without side-effects of any kind. Fortunately, these have been far less sinister than the side-effects associated with traditional medications used to treat the chronic illnesses CBD oil has been shown to impact, making it a safer choice under any circumstances. Better still, the number of people affected by side-effects were relatively small, meaning that not only are the side-effects of CBD oil mild, they are also rare. This chapter will reveal three of the more common symptoms experienced, as well as ways to manage them or even avoid them completely.

Most common side effects

One of the most common side effects of CBD oil is a drop-in blood pressure. In fact, it's a bit of a misnomer to call this a side effect as high blood pressure is one of the conditions CBD oil is recommended for treating. However, since there are numerous other conditions which CBD oil is useful for not all users will have high blood pressure. This means any drop-in blood pressure could affect them in a noticeable way. A common symptom of this is light-headedness. When a heart-healthy person experiences a drop-in blood pressure they may experience slight dizziness or light-headedness. This usually doesn't last long, but it can be significant enough to require the individual to sit down for a moment until the feeling passes. Needless to say, it is recommended that any driving or operating of equipment be suspended during this time in order to avoid any serious injury.

A second side-effect reported with the use of CBD oil is dry mouth. Fortunately, dry mouth is little more than a nuisance, not anything of serious consequence. However, side-effects are side-effects no matter how small and unimportant they may be. The reason behind this symptom is that the Endocannabinoid system is known to reduce production of saliva. Again, this isn't anything that would pose any real threat, like dizziness could in the case of flying a plane, however it is something that might be experienced with high dosages of CBD oil.

The third side-effect that is reported among users of CBD oil is drowsiness. As with the case of low blood pressure, this is less of a side effect and more of an actual use. Since CBD oil is used to combat stress and anxiety, all symptoms of stress and anxiety are also impacted. Insomnia is one such symptom. However, since not all users will be suffering from stress or insomnia any drowsiness may be a problem, especially during the workday. In the case of someone experiencing drowsiness from CBD oil it is recommended that they avoid driving or operating machinery for about half an hour after dosage, long enough for any side effects to wear off.

Treatment strategies

Sometimes a person can't change when they use CBD oil, meaning that they have to perform their normal day-to-day activities in spite of any side-effects that the oil might have. Fortunately, since the side-effects are relatively mild they are also easy to counter. Better still, you don't need extra medications or supplements to negate the side-effects. Instead, some basic foods or beverages can be enough to keep your system in balance, thus reducing or even eliminating any unwanted symptoms altogether.

In the event that you experience dry mouth when taking CBD oil, the obvious solution is to drink extra water when taking the oil. By drinking one or two glasses of water with each dose you will keep your body hydrated, thus eliminating any complications due to dry mouth. Taking CBD oil with meals can also help as your saliva production is increased while eating. This will reduce the impact that the oil has on saliva production, as well as giving you a chance to drink extra liquids in a more natural setting.

The best way to counter a drop-in blood pressure is to raise your blood pressure when taking CBD oil. One way to do this is with exercise. If you can run or perform a cardio workout when ingesting CBD oil, you will avoid any dizziness due to your blood pressure becoming excessively low. If exercise isn't an option you can always drink a caffeinated beverage, such as coffee, soda or an energy drink. This will elevate your blood pressure enough to negate any effects caused by a sudden reduction in pressure due to the CBD oil.

Drowsiness can also be countered with caffeinated beverages. Essentially, feeling sleepy is a symptom of low blood pressure, so any method for countering the effects of reduced blood pressure will also work for drowsiness. Additionally, simple movements such as walking around will help to keep the blood flowing and the drowsiness at bay. Perhaps the most important thing is to avoid anything that might make you feel relaxed, thus increasing the sense of drowsiness. Therefore, avoid comfy sofas and soft, relaxing music while taking CBD oil in order to minimize its

Peter Augustine

sleep-inducing effects.

CONCLUSION

Now that you have read this book you have all the information necessary to know whether or not CBD oil is right for you. Whether you suffer from chronic pain, stress and anxiety, or side-effects from other medications, CBD oil offers benefits that can help relieve and even eliminate your suffering. Furthermore, the low risk nature of CBD oil makes it safe for people of all ages and health conditions, even those predisposed to addictive behavior. Finally, the fact that CBD oil side-effects are as mild as they are rare makes this a good choice for anyone seeking relief from stress, pain or any of the other symptoms and conditions CBD oil has been shown to relieve. Here's hoping that CBD oil brings you the same relief that it has to countless others all around the world!

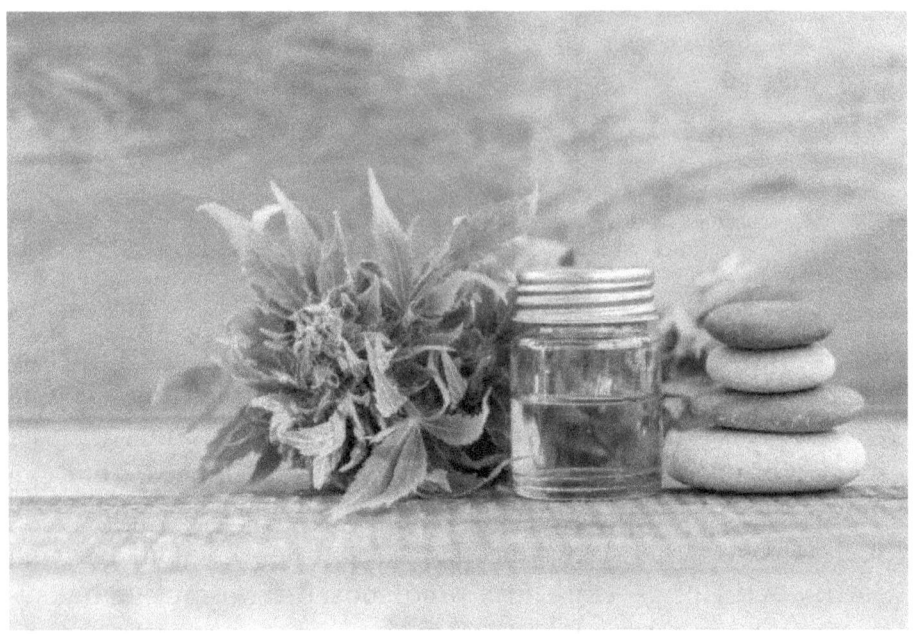

And finally, if you liked the book, I would like to ask you to do me a favor and leave a review for the book on Amazon. Just go to your account on Amazon or click on the link below.

CLICK HERE TO LEAVE A REVIEW ON AMAZON!

Thank you and good luck!